T0209756

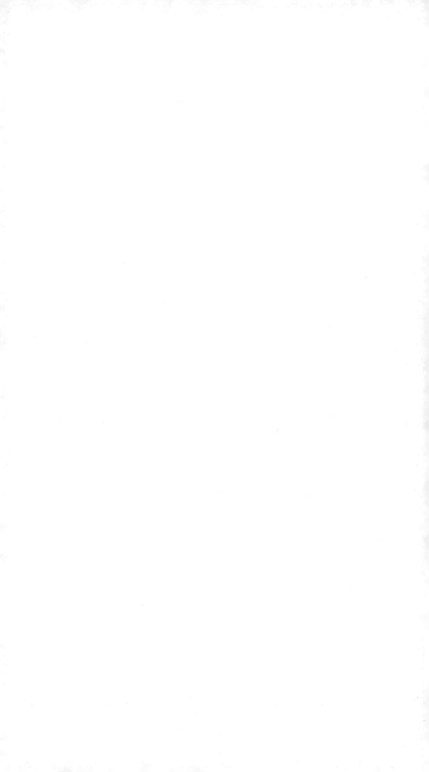

A Word to the Wise

Lessons I learned at 22

Yvonne Faith Russell

WESTBOW
PRESS®
A DIVISION OF THOMAS NELSON
& ZONDERVAN

WestBow Press books may be ordered through
booksellers or by contacting:

WestBow Press
A Division of Thomas Nelson & Zondervan
1663 Liberty Drive
Bloomington, IN 47403
www.westbowpress.com
1 (866) 928-1240

ISBN: 978-1-9736-8095-6 (sc)
ISBN: 978-1-9736-8096-3 (e)

Library of Congress Control Number: 2019919630

Print information available on the last page.

WestBow Press rev. date: 05/01/2020

To my friend, Mia Iaderosa:

This is only the beginning.

Table of Contents

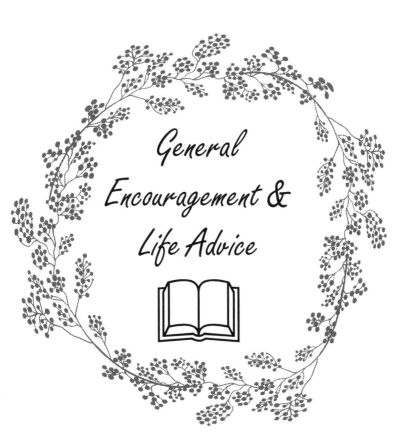

General
Encouragement &
Life Advice

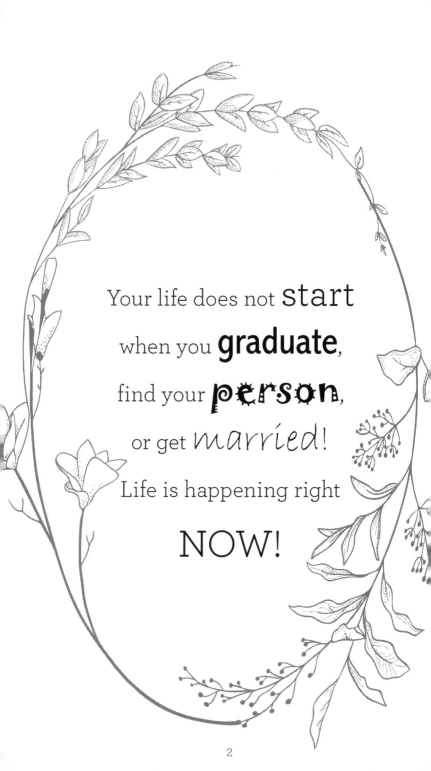

Your life does not start when you **graduate**, find your person, or get *married!* Life is happening right NOW!

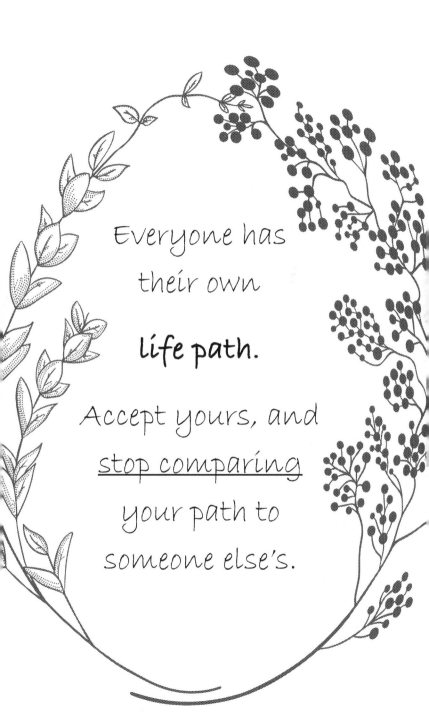

Everyone has
their own

life path.

Accept yours, and
<u>stop comparing</u>
your path to
someone else's.

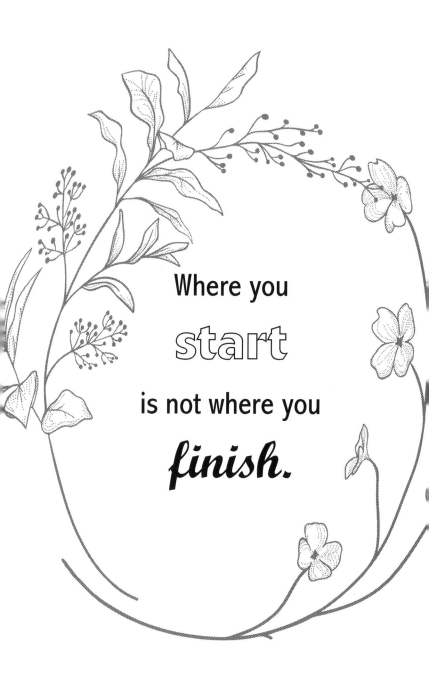

Where you **start** is not where you *finish.*

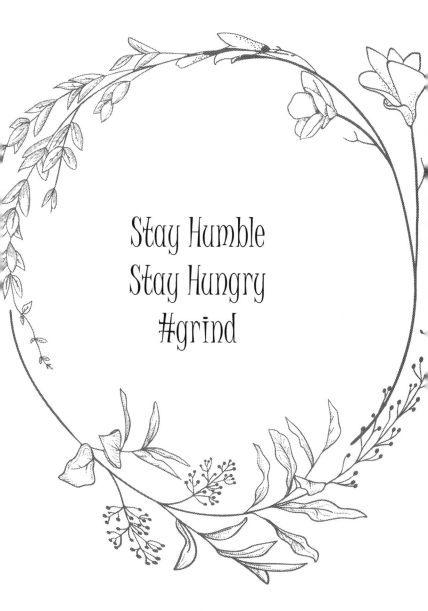

Stay Humble
Stay Hungry
#grind

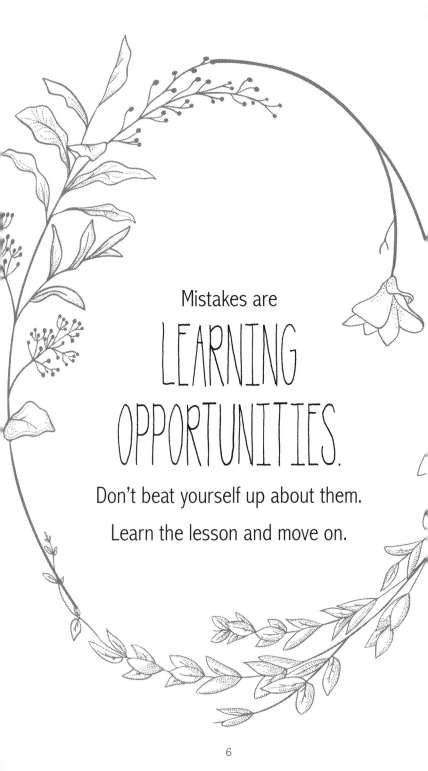

Mistakes are

LEARNING OPPORTUNITIES.

Don't beat yourself up about them.

Learn the lesson and move on.

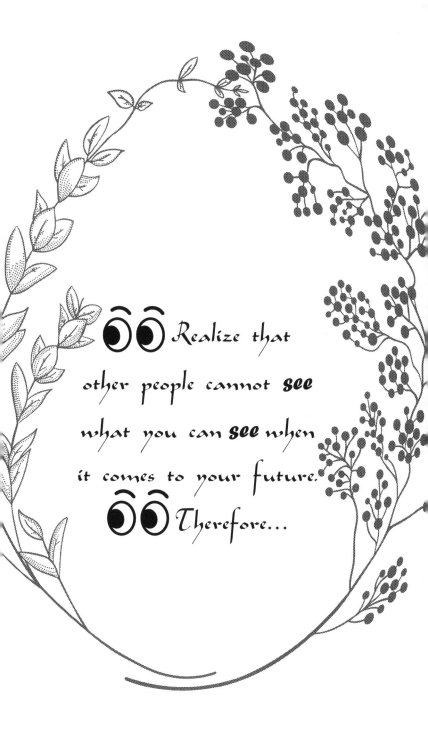

👀 Realize that other people cannot **see** what you can **see** when it comes to your future. 👀 Therefore...

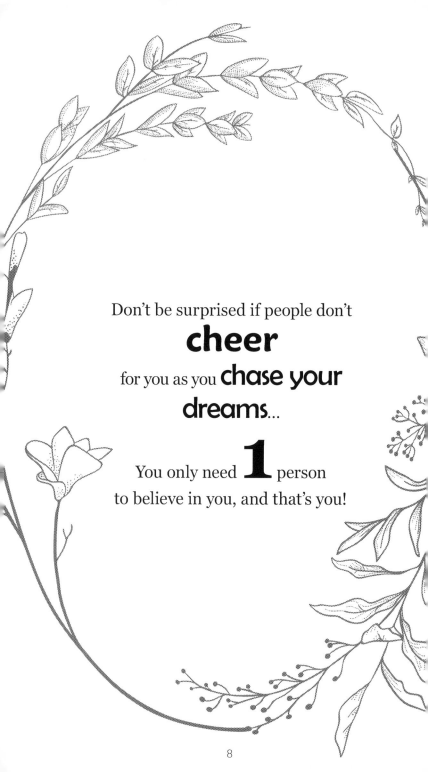

Don't be surprised if people don't
cheer
for you as you **chase your
dreams**...

You only need **1** person
to believe in you, and that's you!

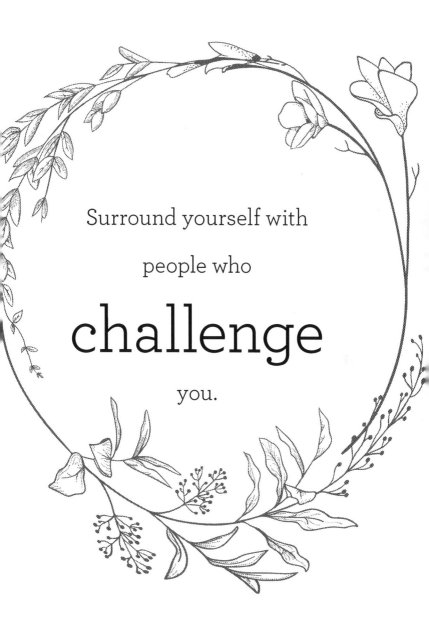

Surround yourself with

people who

challenge

you.

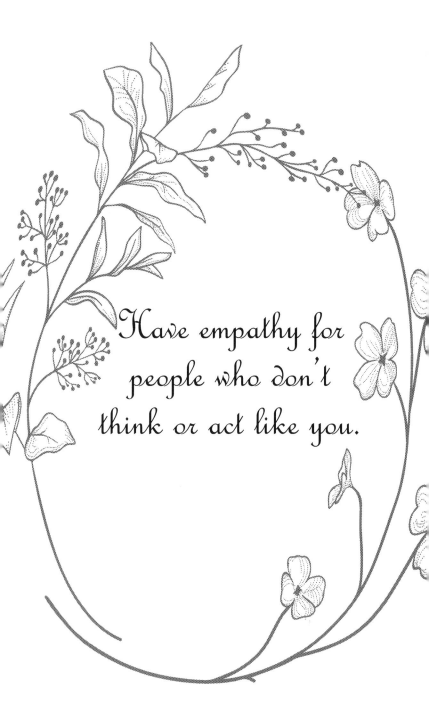

Have empathy for
people who don't
think or act like you.

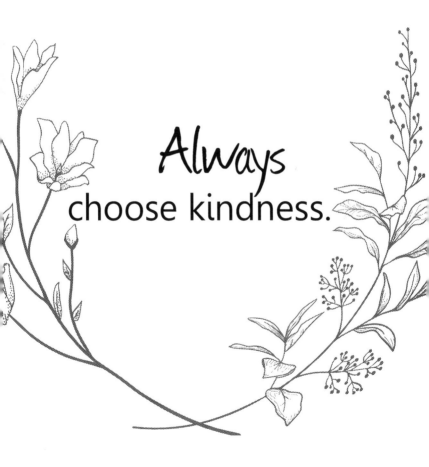

Always
choose kindness.

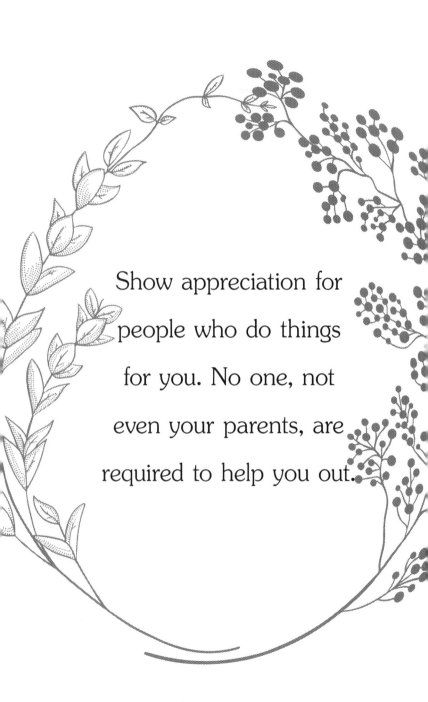

Show appreciation for people who do things for you. No one, not even your parents, are required to help you out.

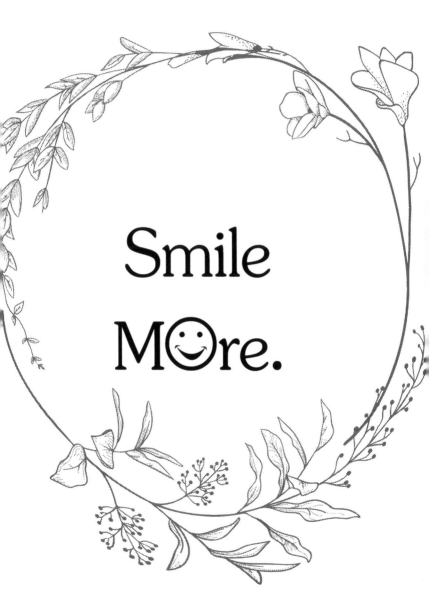

Smile
M☺re.

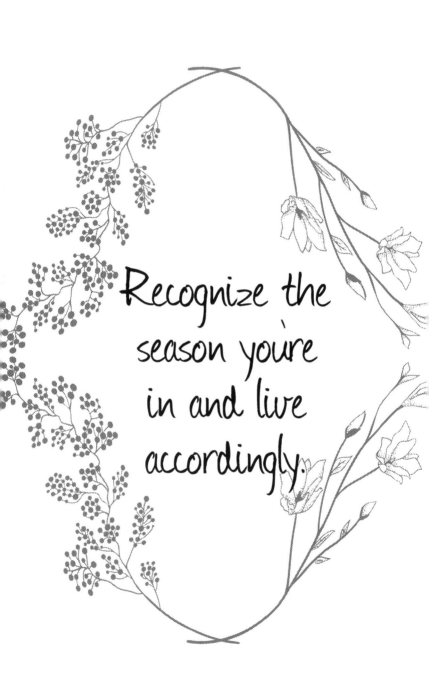

Recognize the
season you're
in and live
accordingly.

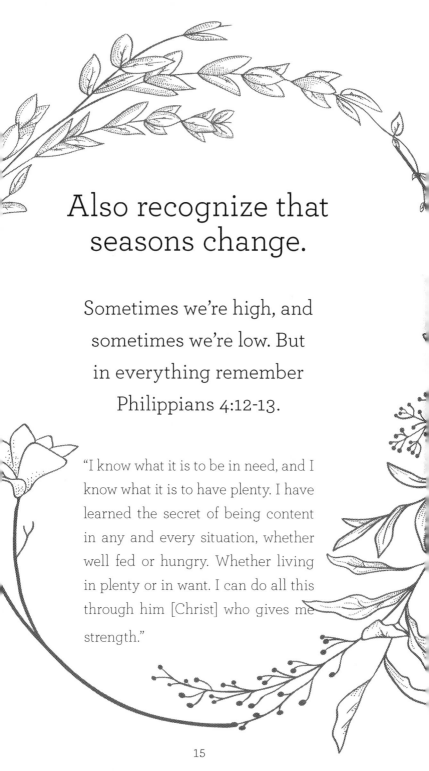

Also recognize that seasons change.

Sometimes we're high, and sometimes we're low. But in everything remember Philippians 4:12-13.

"I know what it is to be in need, and I know what it is to have plenty. I have learned the secret of being content in any and every situation, whether well fed or hungry. Whether living in plenty or in want. I can do all this through him [Christ] who gives me strength."

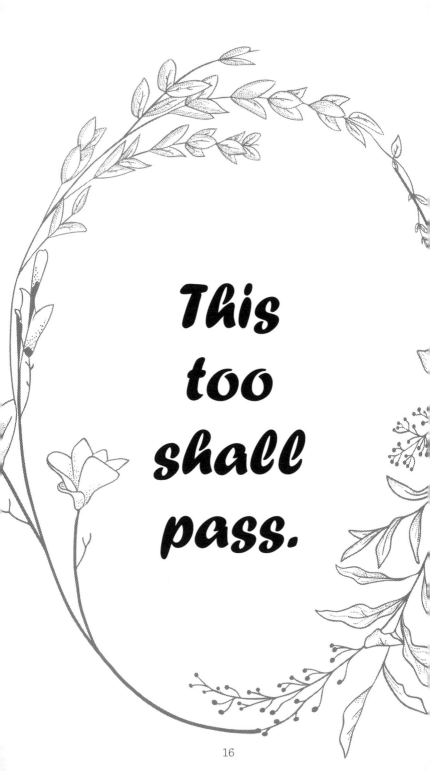

This
too
shall
pass.

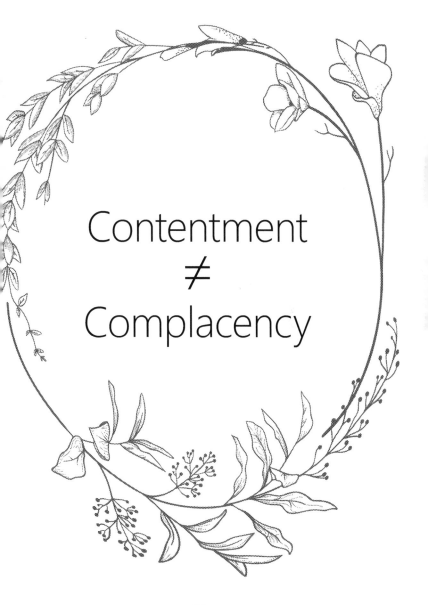

Contentment
≠
Complacency

🚫 Watch for, recognize, and avoid distractions. 👀

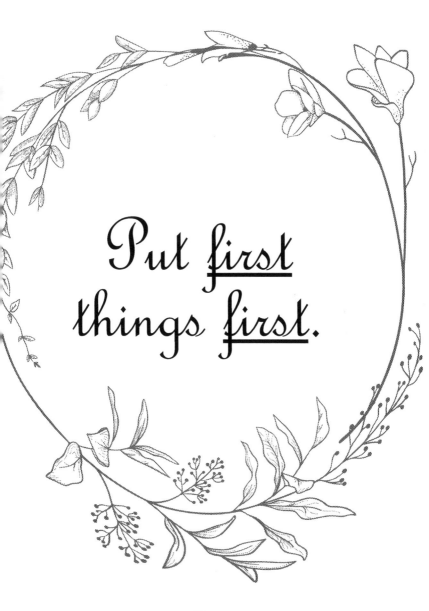

Put *first* things *first*.

Don't **let** college be the BEST years of your *life.*

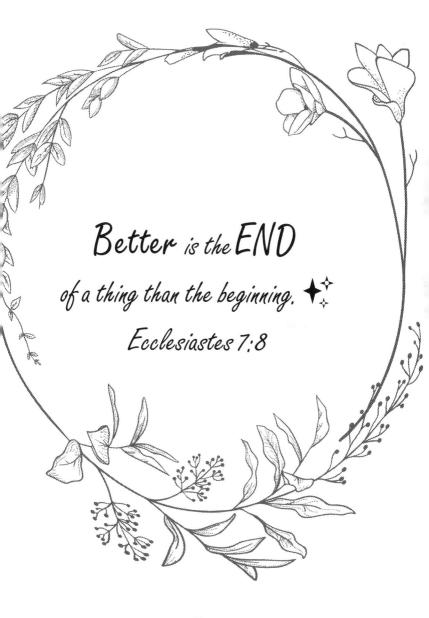

Better is the END
of a thing than the beginning.
Ecclesiastes 7:8

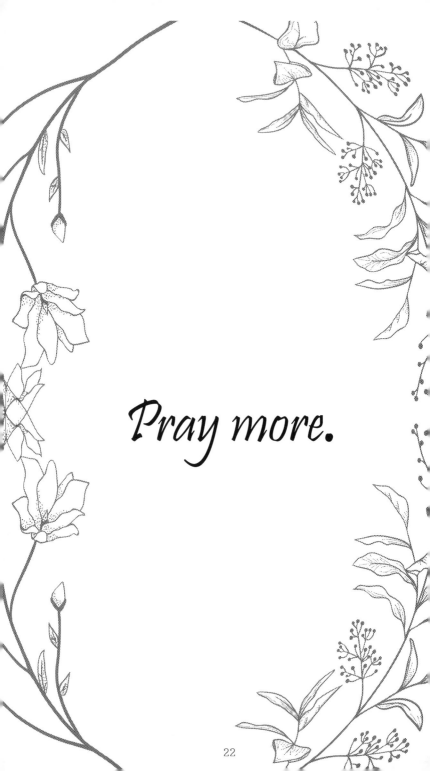

Pray more.

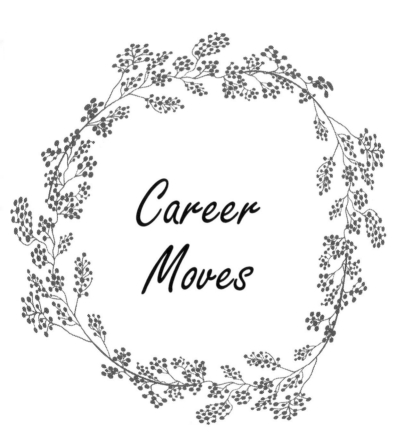

Career
Moves

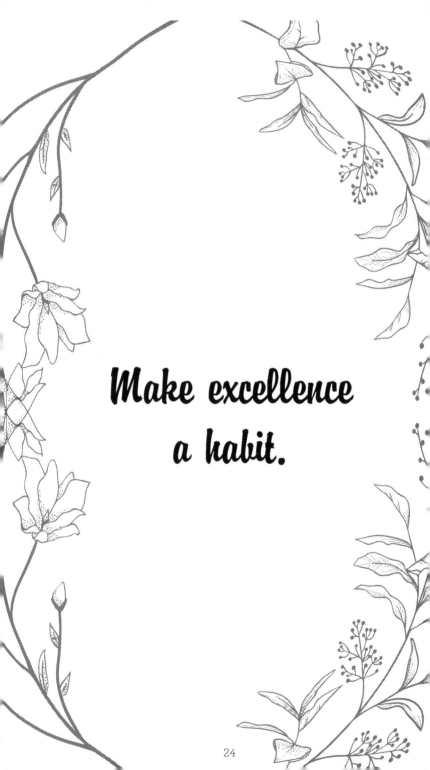

Make excellence
a habit.

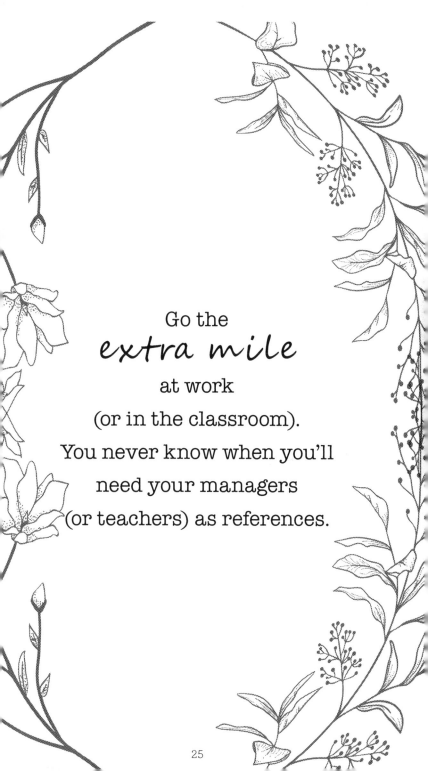

Go the
extra mile
at work
(or in the classroom).
You never know when you'll
need your managers
(or teachers) as references.

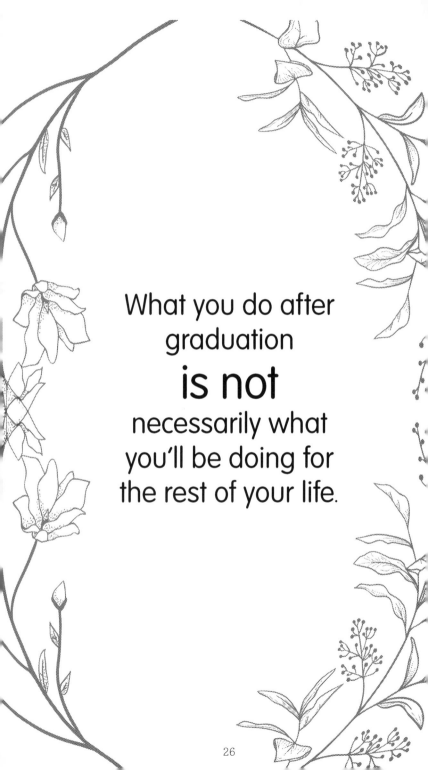

What you do after graduation

is not

necessarily what you'll be doing for the rest of your life.

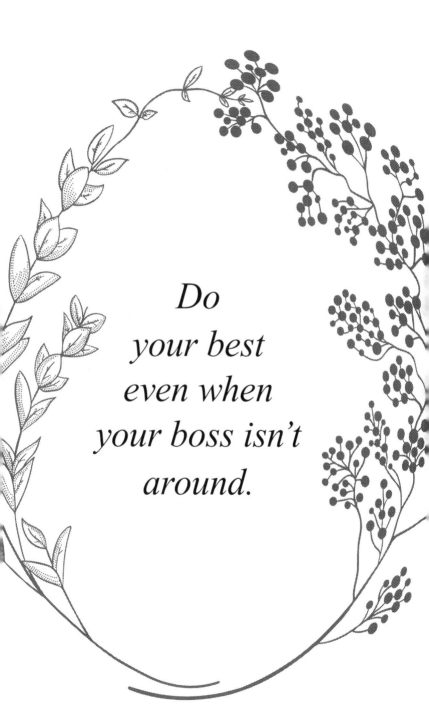

*Do
your best
even when
your boss isn't
around.*

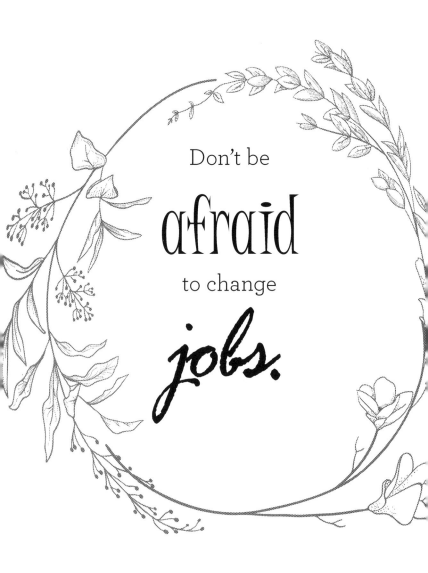

Don't be

afraid

to change

jobs.

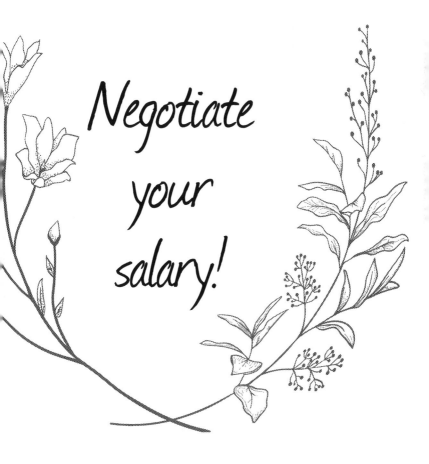

Negotiate your salary!

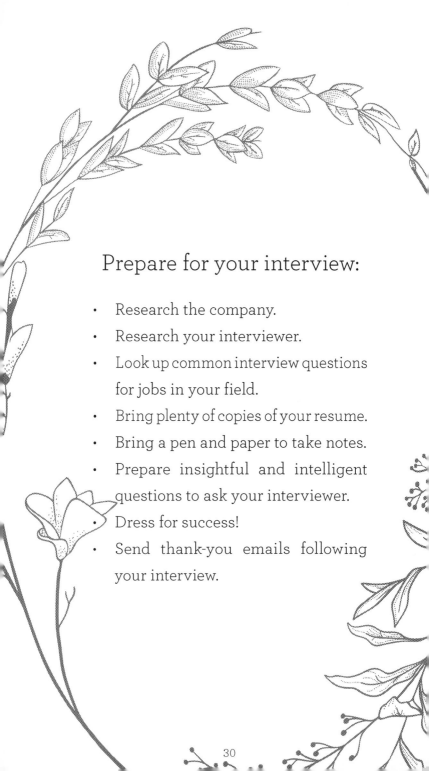

Prepare for your interview:

- Research the company.
- Research your interviewer.
- Look up common interview questions for jobs in your field.
- Bring plenty of copies of your resume.
- Bring a pen and paper to take notes.
- Prepare insightful and intelligent questions to ask your interviewer.
- Dress for success!
- Send thank-you emails following your interview.

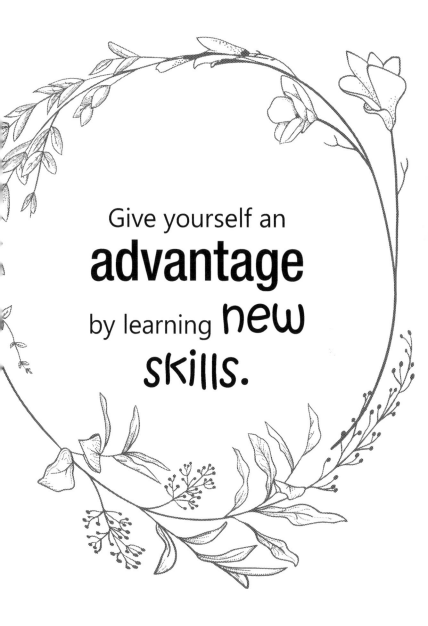

Give yourself an
advantage
by learning new
skills.

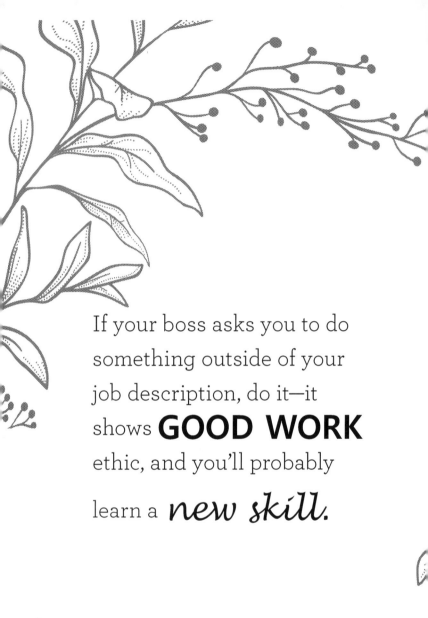

If your boss asks you to do something outside of your job description, do it—it shows **GOOD WORK** ethic, and you'll probably learn a *new skill.*

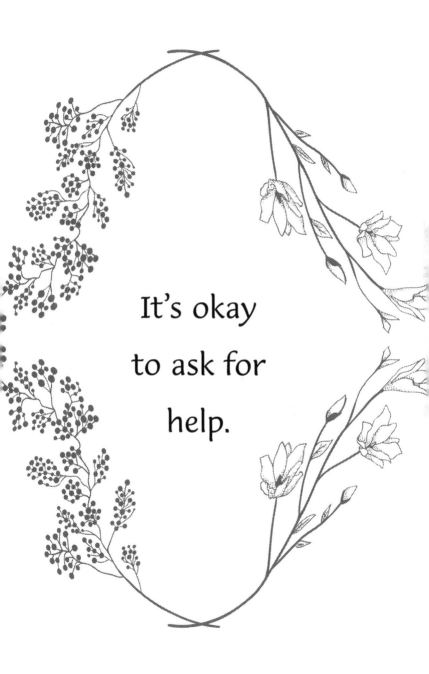

It's okay
to ask for
help.

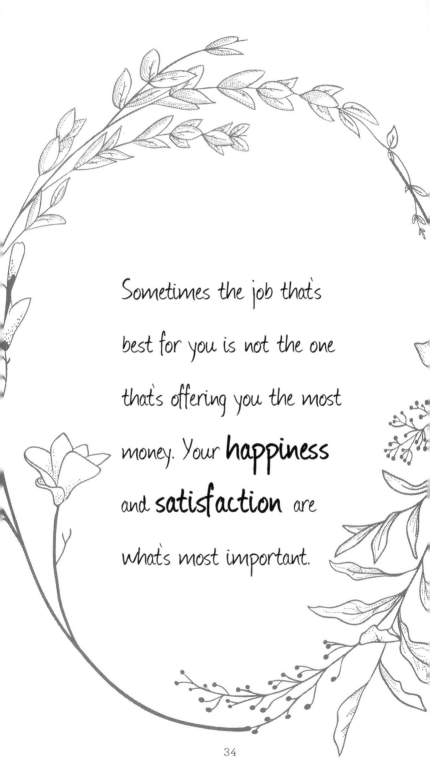

Sometimes the job that's
best for you is not the one
that's offering you the most
money. Your **happiness**
and **satisfaction** are
what's most important.

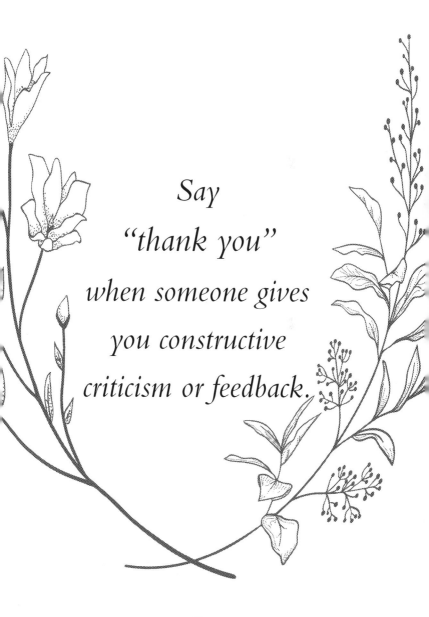

Say
"thank you"
when someone gives
you constructive
criticism or feedback.

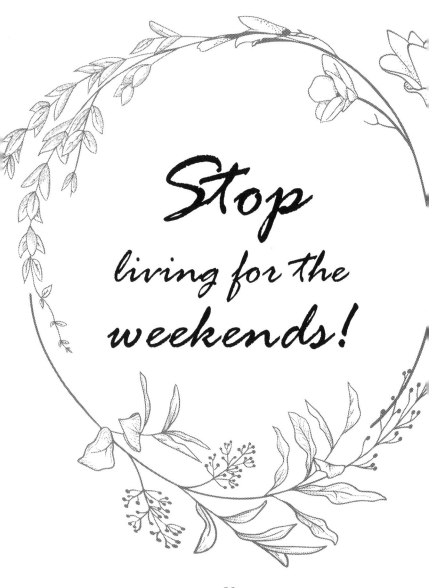

Stop
living for the
weekends!

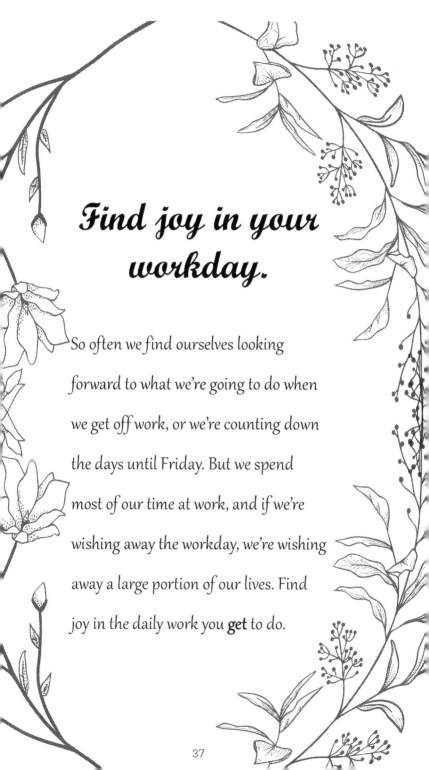

Find joy in your workday.

So often we find ourselves looking forward to what we're going to do when we get off work, or we're counting down the days until Friday. But we spend most of our time at work, and if we're wishing away the workday, we're wishing away a large portion of our lives. Find joy in the daily work you **get** to do.

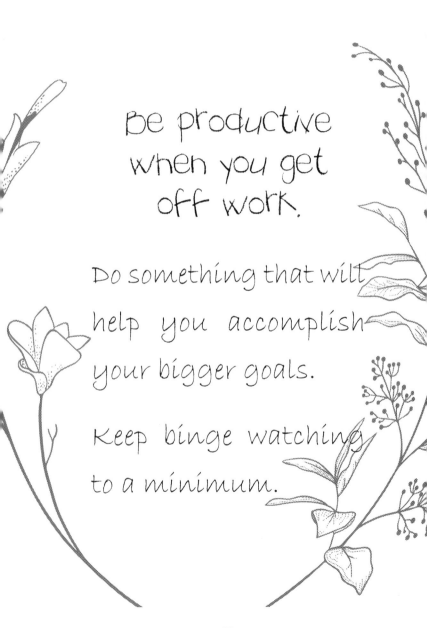

Be productive
when you get
off work.

Do something that will
help you accomplish
your bigger goals.

Keep binge watching
to a minimum.

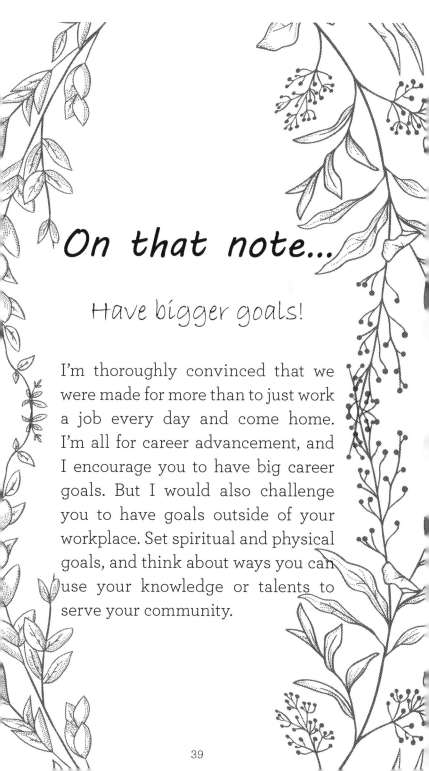

On that note...

Have bigger goals!

I'm thoroughly convinced that we were made for more than to just work a job every day and come home. I'm all for career advancement, and I encourage you to have big career goals. But I would also challenge you to have goals outside of your workplace. Set spiritual and physical goals, and think about ways you can use your knowledge or talents to serve your community.

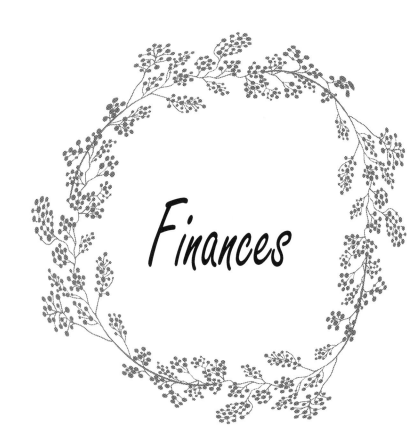

Finances

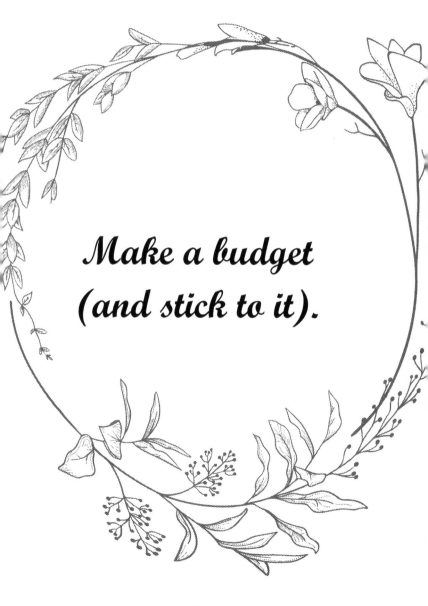

Make a budget
(and stick to it).

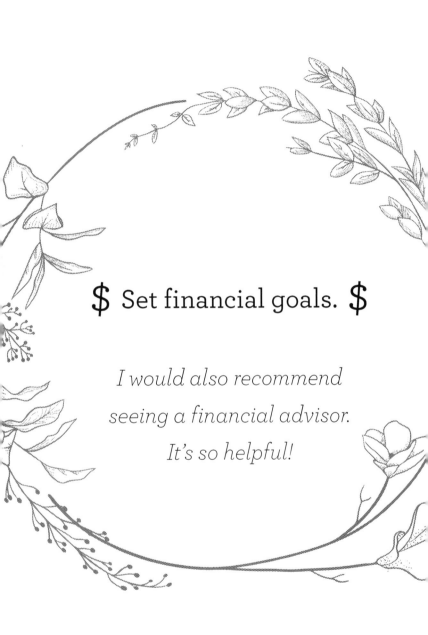

$ Set financial goals. $

I would also recommend
seeing a financial advisor.
It's so helpful!

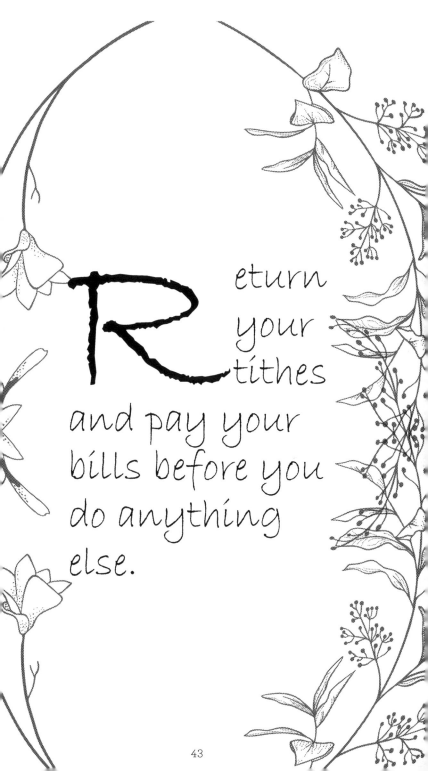

Return your tithes and pay your bills before you do anything else.

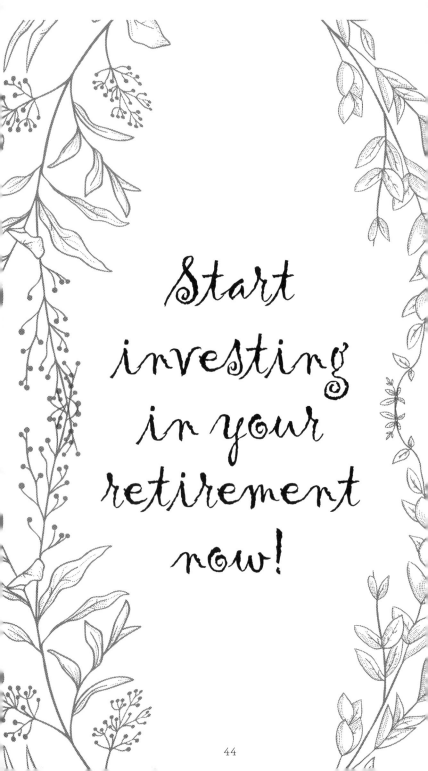

Start investing in your retirement now!

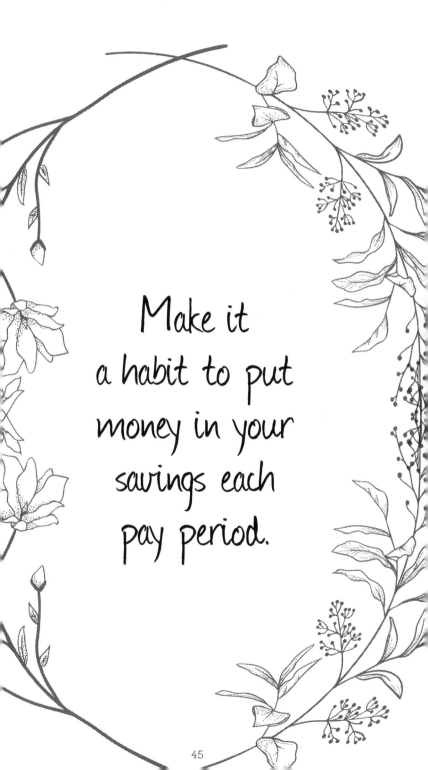

Make it
a habit to put
money in your
savings each
pay period.

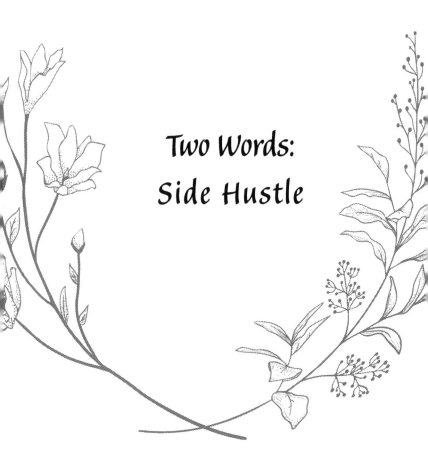

Two Words:
Side Hustle

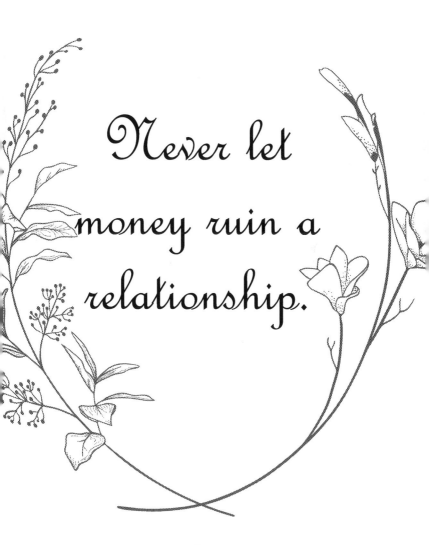

Never let
money ruin a
relationship.

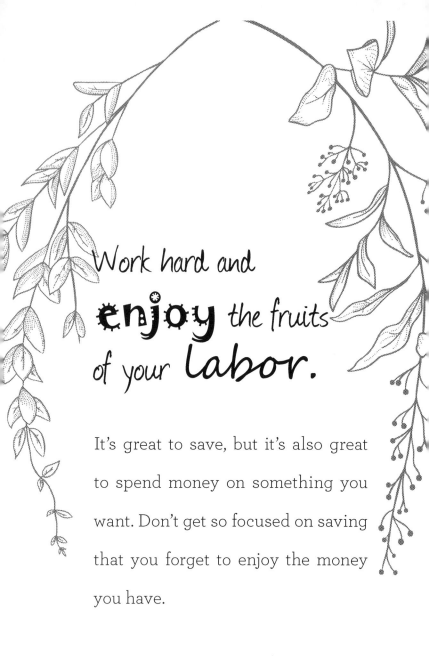

Work hard and **enjoy** the fruits of your **labor.**

It's great to save, but it's also great to spend money on something you want. Don't get so focused on saving that you forget to enjoy the money you have.

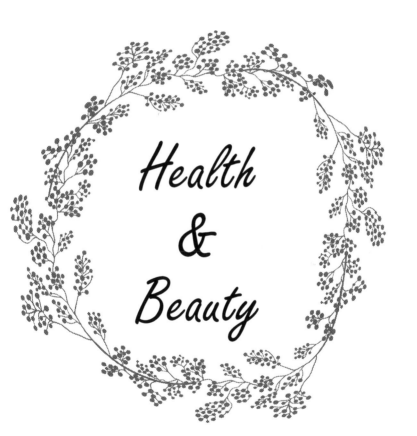

Health
&
Beauty

Invest in your health.

Do what you need to do to stay healthy both physically and mentally. Start getting massages, see a dietician, chiropractor, therapist, counselor, or whatever specialist you may need. Take a vitamin, exercise, get some sleep, and take a sick day if you need it— that's what they're there for! These investments might be a few more expenses in your budget, but that's why it's called an investment! I promise it will be worth it once you see how good you start feeling.

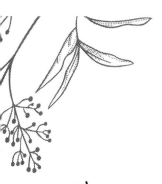

Use your vacation days.

Regular breaks help you avoid burnout.

Even if you're unable to take a weeklong vacation, it's still important to take some time off work. Maximize your vacation days by taking off the days before or after a long weekend. You can take a road trip to visit friends or relax right where you are. You don't have to go somewhere exotic to rest and regroup.

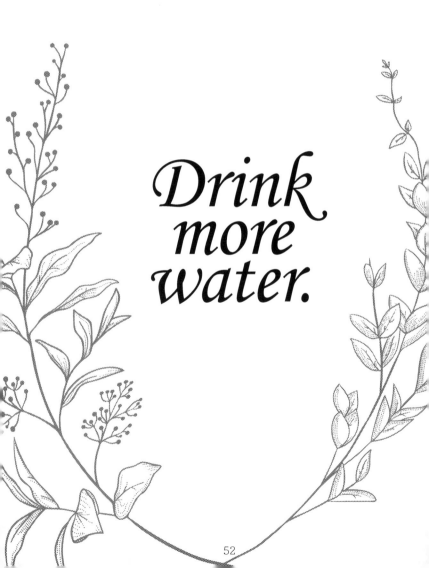

Drink
more
water.

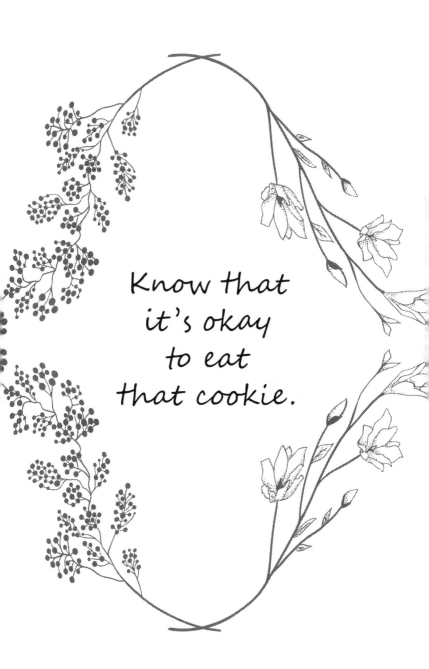

Know that
it's okay
to eat
that cookie.

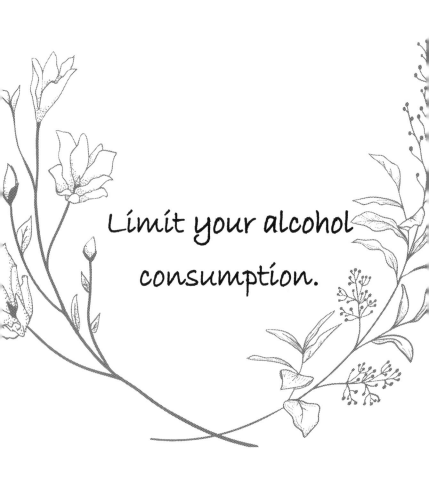

Limit your alcohol consumption.

Develop a good

skin care routine.

African Black Soap and

Witch Hazel y'all...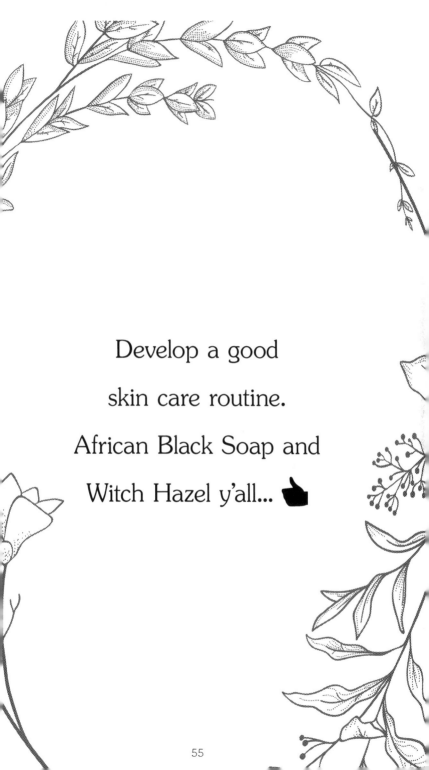

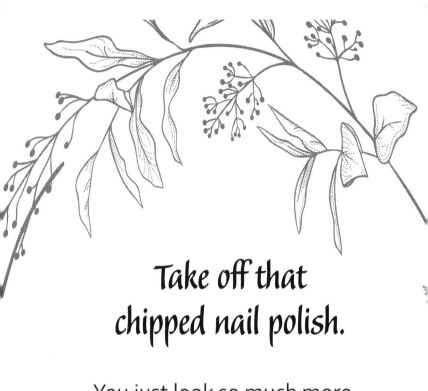

Take off that chipped nail polish.

You just look so much more put together if your nails are either painted or not. The chipped look only worked in grade school (and even then, it didn't).

Start anti-aging treatments now in your early 20's.

There's no way to truly reverse wrinkles, but if you start taking preventative measures now, your skin will be looking younger, longer. ♡

Remember that personality > looks.

Don't get me wrong, I love to look cute, and there's nothing wrong with that or caring about your appearance. But don't be that girl that's made up from top to bottom but has no personality.

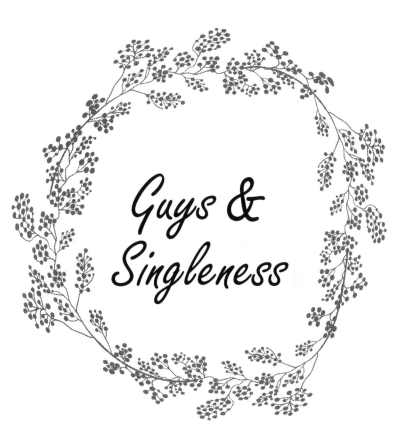

Guys &
Singleness

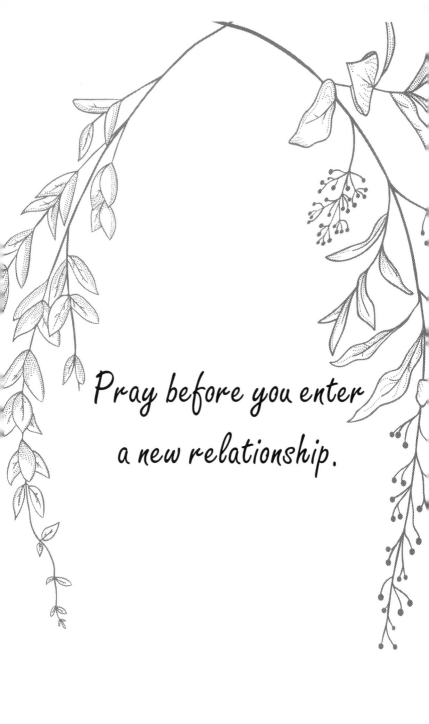

Pray before you enter
a new relationship.

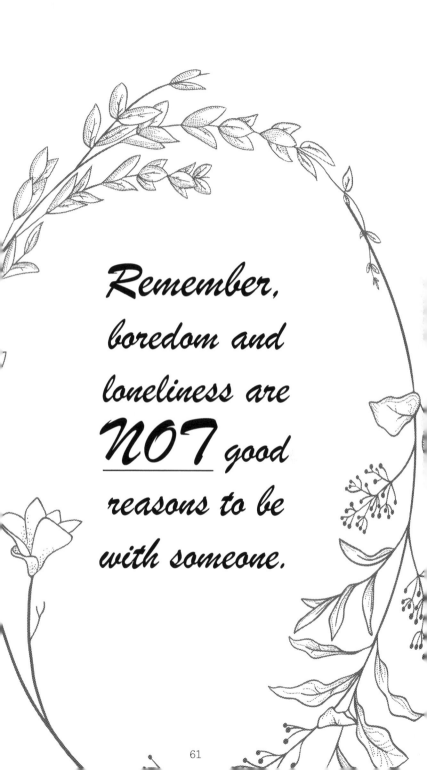

Remember, boredom and loneliness are **NOT** good reasons to be with someone.

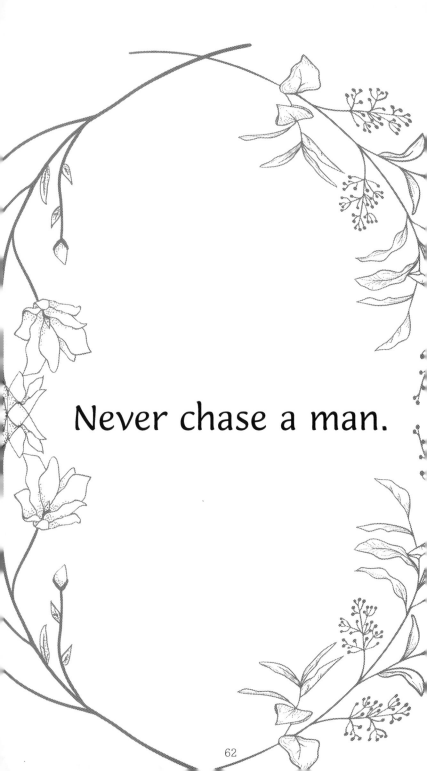

Never chase a man.

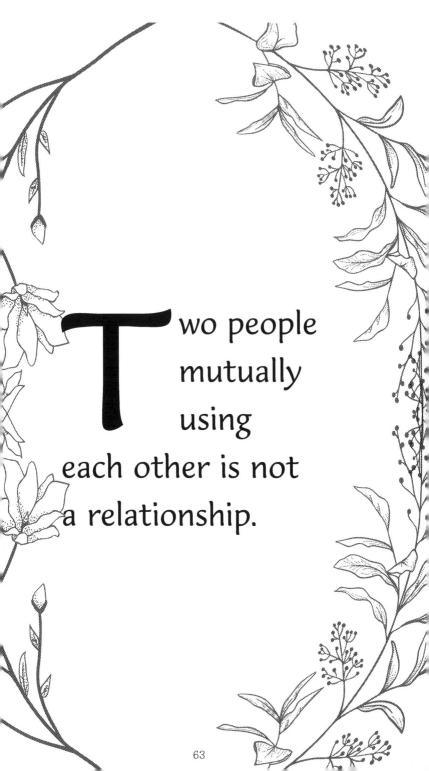

Two people
mutually
using
each other is not
a relationship.

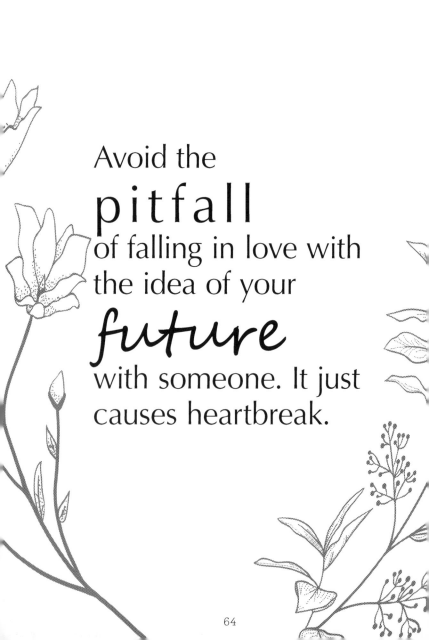

Avoid the **pitfall** of falling in love with the idea of your *future* with someone. It just causes heartbreak.

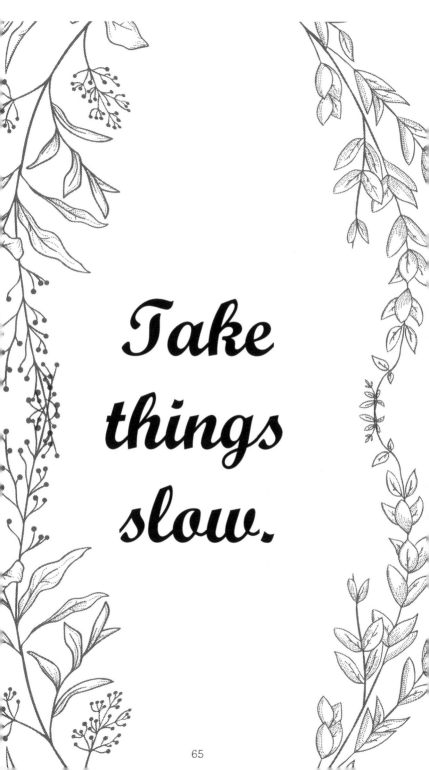

Take things slow.

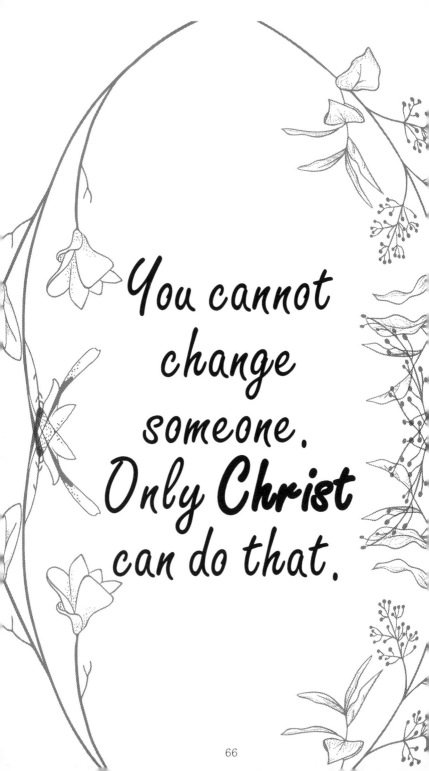

You cannot change someone.
Only **Christ** can do that.

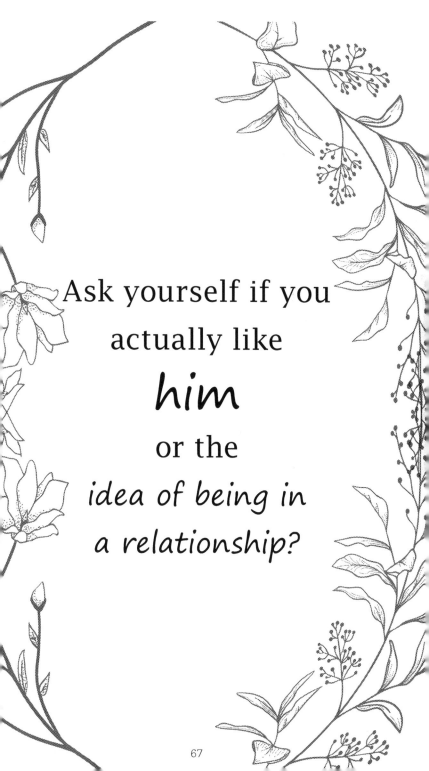

Ask yourself if you
actually like

him

or the

*idea of being in
a relationship?*

Also ask yourself if you actually like *him* or the **way he makes you feel**?

This is a tricky one because you should definitely be with someone who makes you feel good and amazing, but sometimes it's hard to differentiate between if we actually like the man or the way he makes us feel physically or emotionally. Your guy should encourage you, but you shouldn't need him to shower you with compliments all the time for you to feel good about yourself. Your self-worth comes from Christ.

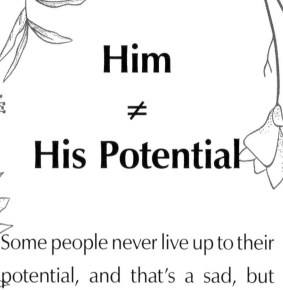

Him

≠

His Potential

Some people never live up to their potential, and that's a sad, but true, fact. I believe in investing in people, and I love giving people the benefit of the doubt. But sometimes you just have to take people for what they are and not for what they could be.

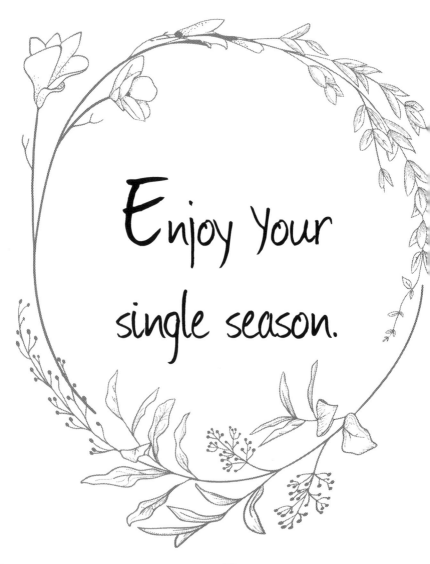

Enjoy Your single season.

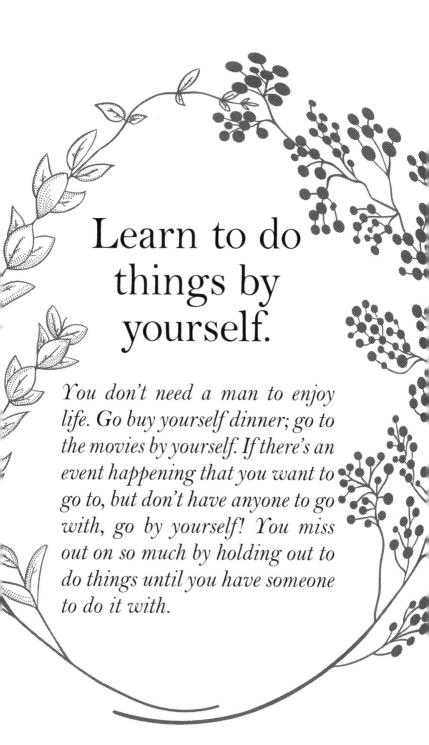

Learn to do things by yourself.

You don't need a man to enjoy life. Go buy yourself dinner; go to the movies by yourself. If there's an event happening that you want to go to, but don't have anyone to go with, go by yourself! You miss out on so much by holding out to do things until you have someone to do it with.

Realize that God, not a man, is your provider.

God does not want any man to take His place in your life. In modern society, many women (and I've been here too) look to a man to support them financially (buying nice gifts, giving money for the nail salon, filling up the gas tank, paying for meals, etc.). But God doesn't want another man to do His job. He is our source. God has blessed me financially (and He wants to bless you too) so that those things don't impress me anymore. I can take myself out to dinner and buy my own flowers (although it's still really nice coming from a man, I'm not going to lie). The more independent I become (by staying dependent on God), the less I'm woo'd by these displays of provision, and the more I can think critically and determine if I like the guy himself or the things he's doing for me.

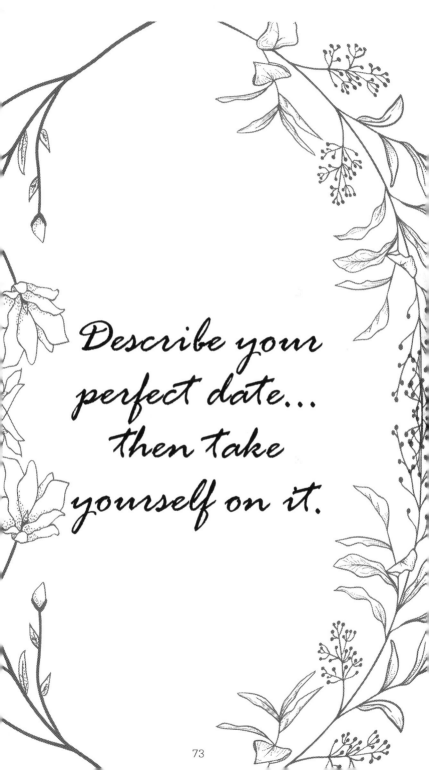

Describe your
perfect date...
then take
yourself on it.

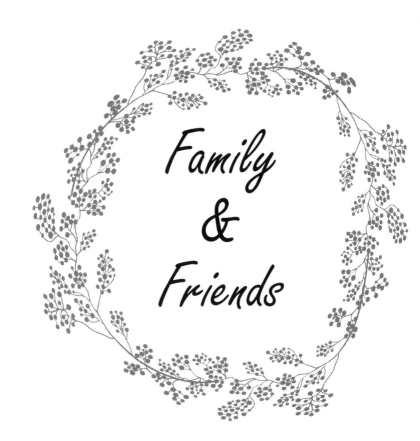

Family
&
Friends

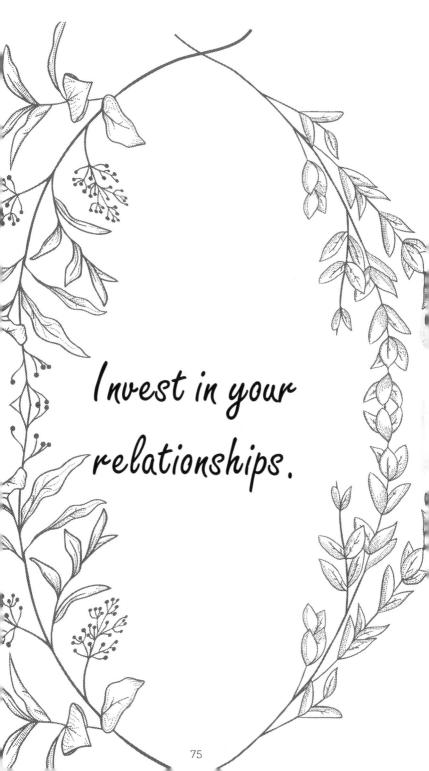

Invest in your relationships.

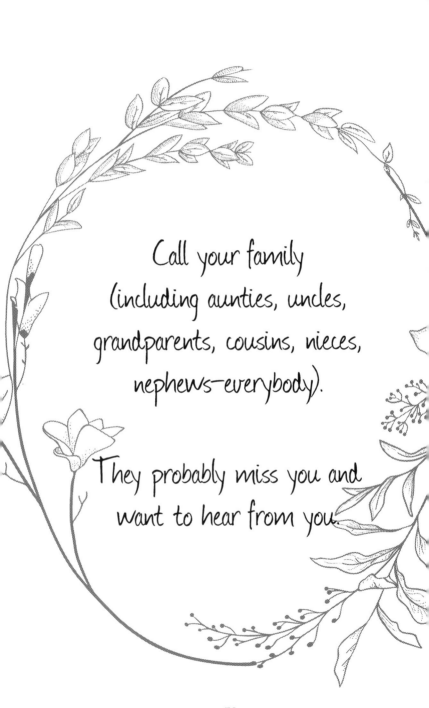

Call your family
(including aunties, uncles,
grandparents, cousins, nieces,
nephews—everybody).

They probably miss you and
want to hear from you.

Realize that your parents are human too, so extend grace to them.

Our parents are people just like us. They don't have all the answers, they've made mistakes, they have flaws, they've disappointed us, they've maybe hurt our feelings, but that's part of being human. Forgive them like you would anyone else and overlook their character flaws. God has extended grace to us, and we ought to extend grace to others, especially our parents.

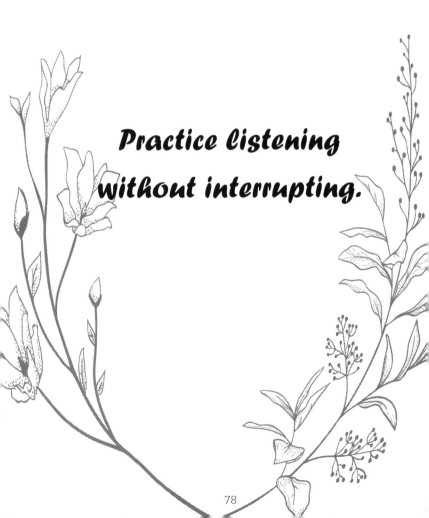

Practice listening without interrupting.

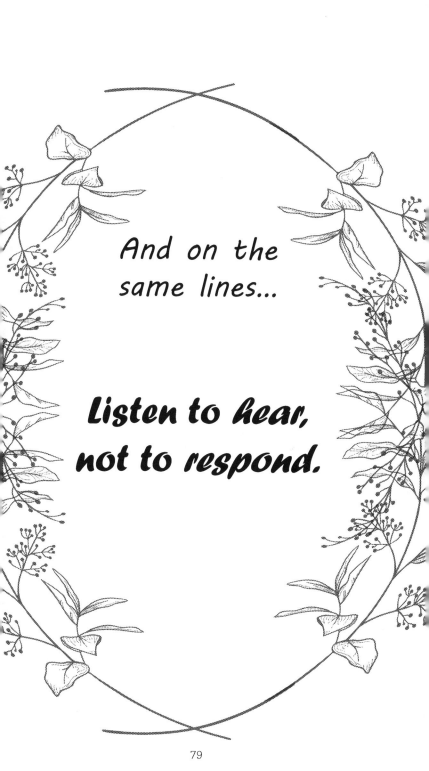

And on the
same lines...

**Listen to hear,
not to respond.**

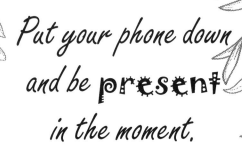

Put your phone down and be present *in the moment.*

Everything does not have to be documented on social media. If you're with someone, let that be enough; give them your attention. If you're constantly looking at your screen, you're sending the message that your phone is more important than they are.

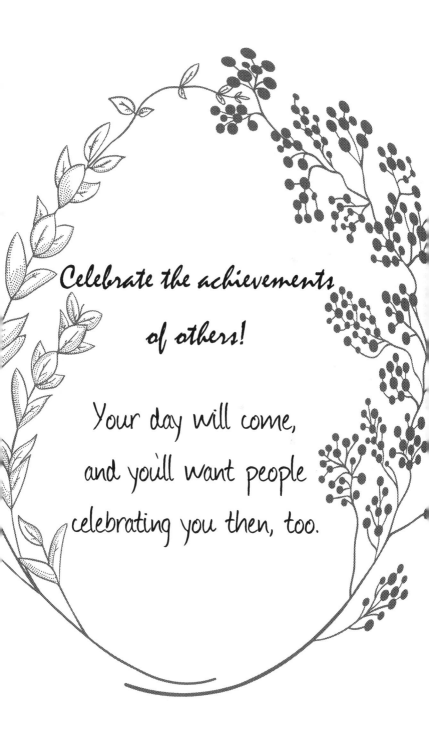

Celebrate the achievements
of others!

Your day will come,
and you'll want people
celebrating you then, too.

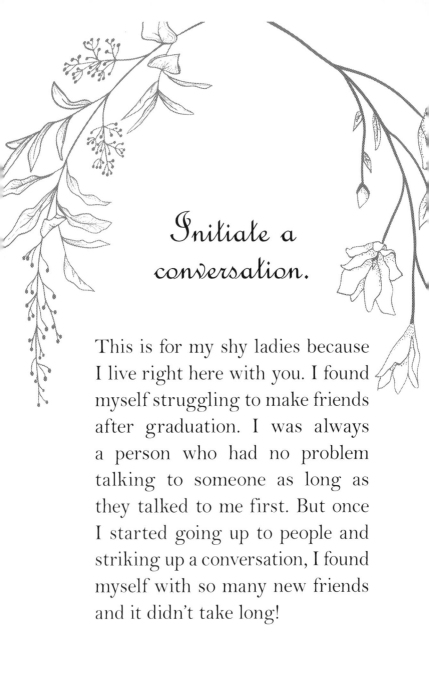

Initiate a conversation.

This is for my shy ladies because I live right here with you. I found myself struggling to make friends after graduation. I was always a person who had no problem talking to someone as long as they talked to me first. But once I started going up to people and striking up a conversation, I found myself with so many new friends and it didn't take long!

Become a YES person.

Another one for the introverts here. Don't get me wrong, I love my alone time and staying in to watch Netflix and eat pizza on a Friday night, but there is so much to gain by saying yes to different social events. You meet so many new people and end up at places and events you might not have ordinarily been. You also establish deeper connections with people by spending time with them outside of the sphere in which you normally meet. Plus, if you actually show up instead of cancelling, people will invite you to more things.

Take a step back and think about how different people in your life might see you.

Do your co-workers see you as a negative Nellie or someone who's always in a great mood? Do your parents see you as an ungrateful child or a compassionate daughter? Do your supervisors/professors see you as a lazy worker/student or do they see you as a young woman with great work ethic?

If the view is negative, consider making adjustments.

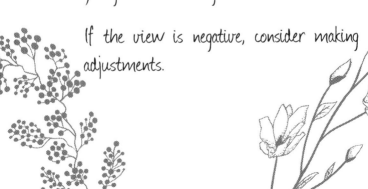

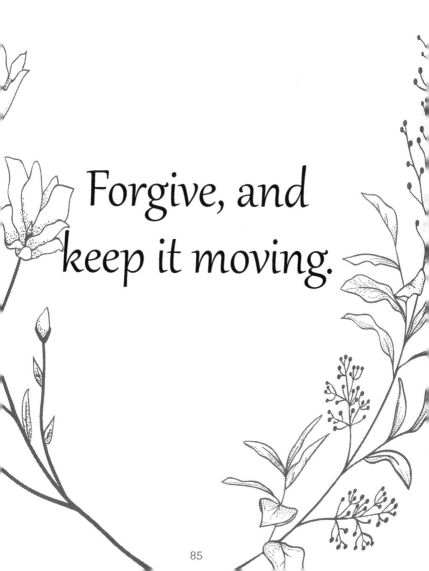

Forgive, and
keep it moving.

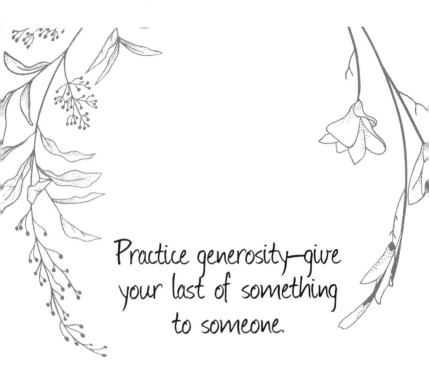

Practice generosity—give
your last of something
to someone.

This can be a K-cup, piece of gum,
dollar bill, favorite drink you keep
stashed away in your drawer, whatever! The
point is to be a little selfless here. People
might forget what exactly you gave them,
but they will remember your attitude and
willingness to give.

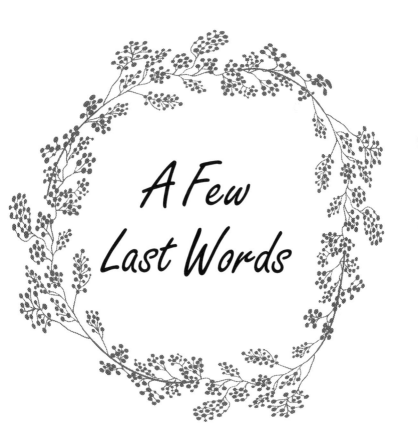

A Few
Last Words

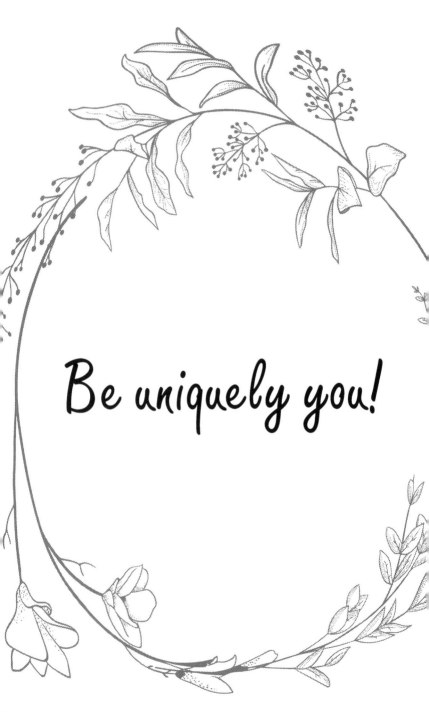

Be uniquely you!

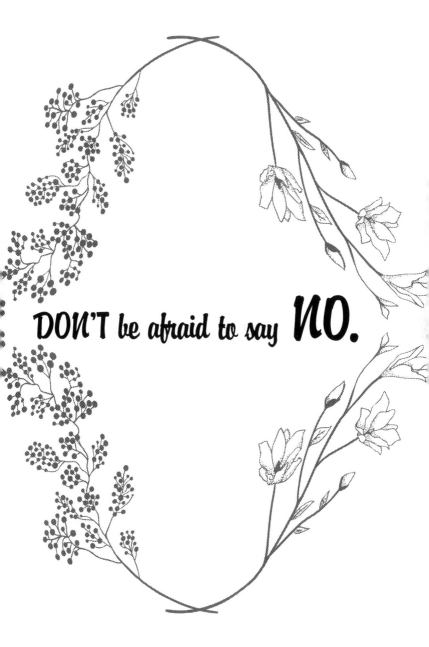

DON'T be afraid to say NO.

Take time to self-reflect.

Why are you upset? Are you really afraid or hurt? Ask yourself the tough questions, and you'll be surprised at what you learn about yourself.

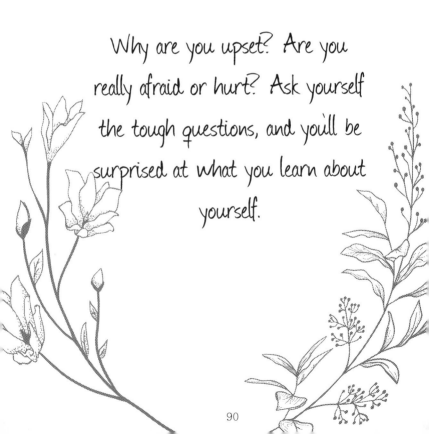

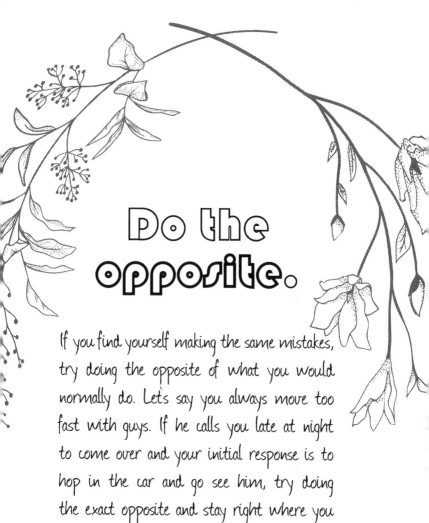

Do the opposite.

If you find yourself making the same mistakes, try doing the opposite of what you would normally do. Let's say you always move too fast with guys. If he calls you late at night to come over and your initial response is to hop in the car and go see him, try doing the exact opposite and stay right where you are. You know what's going to happen when you come over and you can save yourself the temptation. We can only get better results if we start making better decisions.

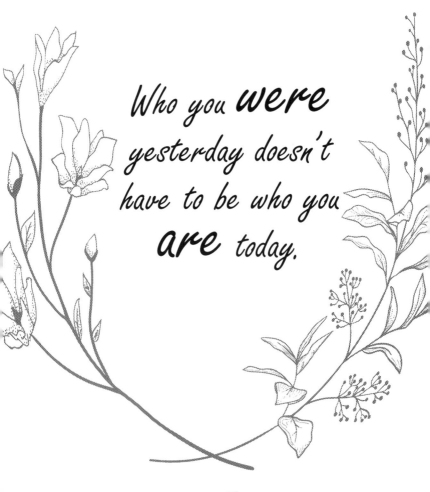

Who you **were** yesterday doesn't have to be who you **are** today.

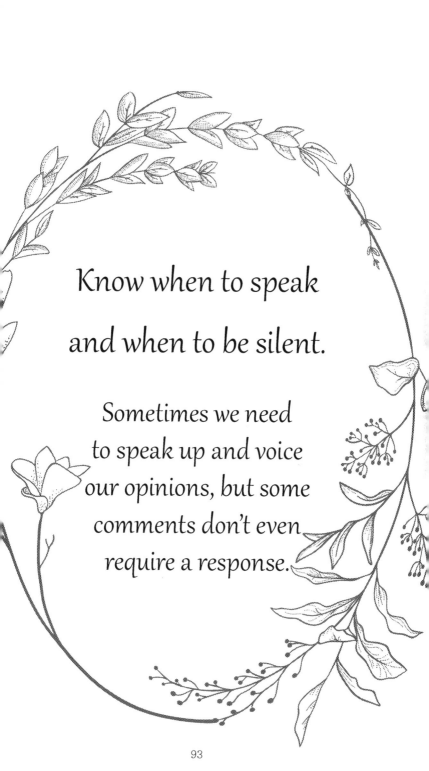

Know when to speak
and when to be silent.

Sometimes we need
to speak up and voice
our opinions, but some
comments don't even
require a response.

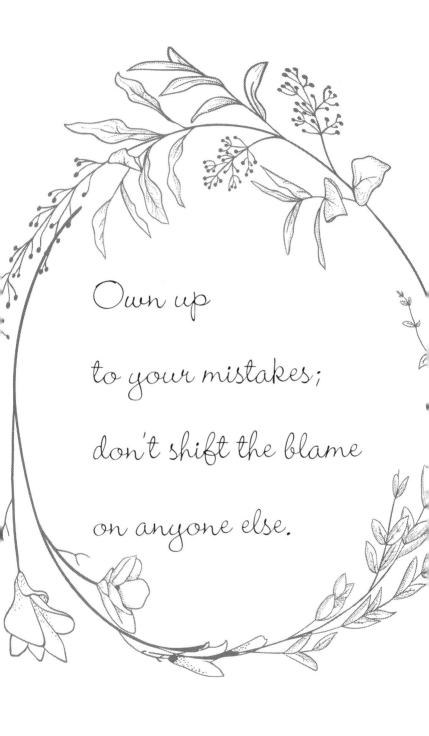

Own up
to your mistakes;
don't shift the blame
on anyone else.

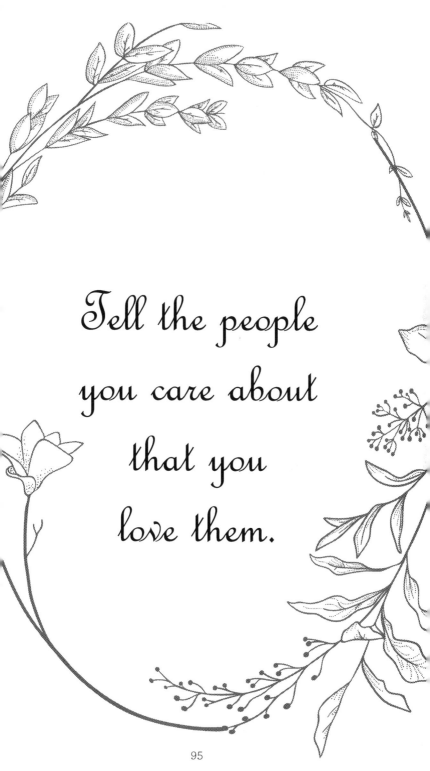

Tell the people
you care about
that you
love them.

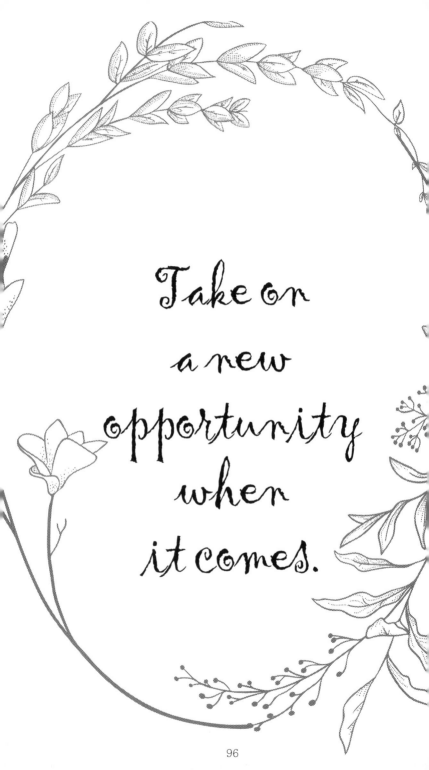

Take on
a new
opportunity
when
it comes.

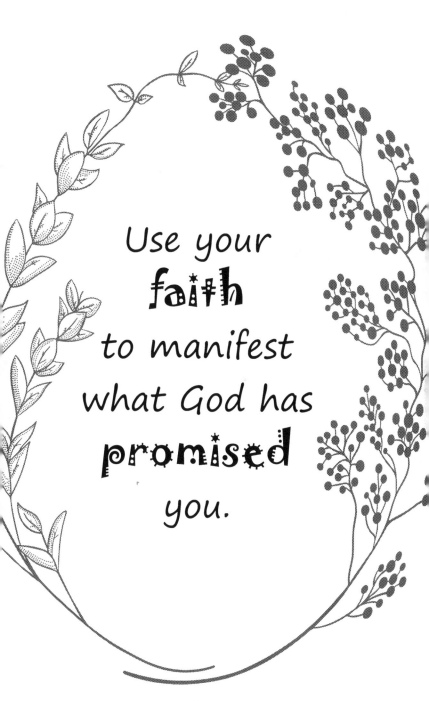

Use your **faith** to manifest what God has **promised** you.

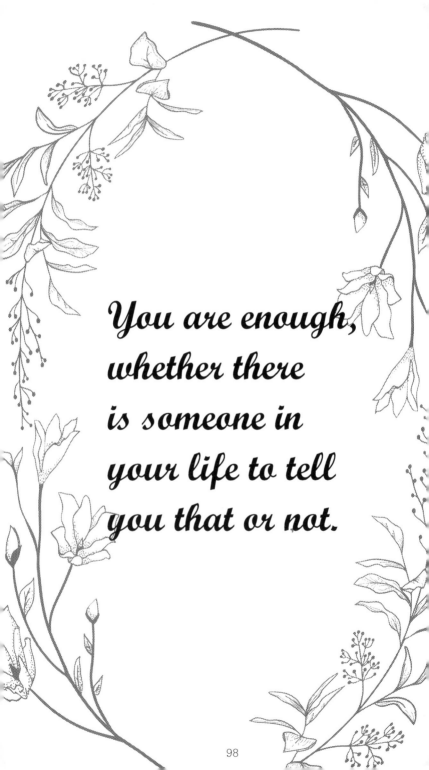

You are enough, whether there is someone in your life to tell you that or not.

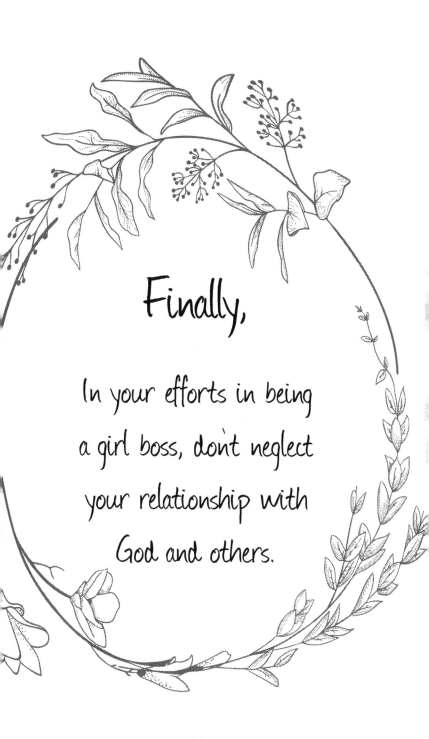

Finally,

In your efforts in being
a girl boss, don't neglect
your relationship with
God and others.

Printed in the United States
By Bookmasters